Fit and fun™

For Life

Liz Caldwell
and Barry Siff

PEAK SPORTSpress®
Boulder, Colorado

Fit and Fun™ for Life

Before embarking on any exercise program, including the exercises included in this book, everyone with a know heart or blood-pressure condition, should be examined by a physician.

Printed in the United States of America.

10 9 8 7 6 5 4 3 2 1

Distributed in the United States and Canada by Publishers Group West.

International Standard Book Number: 1-931382-40-9

PEAK SPORTS press®

Peak Sports Press®, an imprint of VeloPress®
1830 North 55th Street
Boulder, Colorado 80301–2700 USA
303/440-0601 • Fax 303/444-6788
E-mail: peaksportspress@7dogs.com

To purchase additional copies of this book or other Peak Sports Press® or VeloPress® books, call 800/234-8356 or visit us on the Web at velopress.com.

Cover and interior design and composition by Rebecca Finkel, F + P Design, Inc.

To all the people

who have played with us

over the years.

Credits

page xi	Liz and Barry, photo by Susan Candee
page 6	Scotch, photo courtesy of the authors
page 10	Abe Kukawka, photo courtesy of Michelle Streif
page 16	Tai Chi, photo by Christopher Wilson
page 31	Disc Golf, photo by Brian Sullivan, Disclife.com
page 34	Boulder Cruisers, photo courtesy of Boulder Cruisers
page 36	Muddy Buddy, photo courtesy of Todd Fields
page 39	Lacrosse Coaching, photo courtesy of the authors
page 50	Bike Polo, photo courtesy of U.S. Bike Polo Association
page 59	Skijoring, photo courtesy of www.skijornow.com
page 60–61	Strength Exercises, photos courtesy of the authors
page 63	Yoga Poses, photos by Öm Time, Boulder
page 65	Net Footbagging, photo courtesy of International Footbag Players Association

Contents

Preface: Our Stories

Liz's Story

Like many people, I put on a few pounds (okay, more than a few) during college. Less activity, more studying, and certainly more partying all conspired against me and the weight added up. It wasn't until after college, while at my first real job, that friends talked me into running with them during our lunch hour.

Soon I was running in races, starting with 5K runs and building to much longer races. In 1982, at my boyfriend's urging, I trained for and did my first triathlon. That was the beginning of nearly ten years of very regimented training, culminating in Ironman distance triathlons. Since I was single, and had a certain amount of job flexibility, training during those ten years was a wonderful social outlet—all of my friends were training, too!

In 1993, with a new Ph.D., a new job, a new husband, and a new baby (in that order!) something started to change. Dedication to that kind of training requires a certain lack of flexibility—in what you eat and drink, when you sleep, and what you do on the weekend. I'd had enough. My rigid lifestyle just didn't make sense any more, and frankly, it wasn't fun. I love to work out, but I was ready for a change. I wanted my activities to be more spontaneous and natural.

Training for adventure racing offers me that kind of fun. I've learned to simply stay active—every day. I enjoy learning new skills, and challenging myself constantly, whether it's by trying my son's skateboard or going for a hike. It's all fun!

Barry's Story

I had played competitive tennis since age 13 (thanks to a push from my older brother) and was co-captain of my college tennis team. For several years after graduation, I continued playing tennis. In the late summer of 1981, I was inspired by a newspaper story to begin running, and I completed my first marathon that fall. I really loved getting out there and running around the beautiful lakes of the northern Detroit suburbs. Five years later, and after probably ten or fifteen more marathons, I discovered triathlons and went to see two friends complete the Hawaii Ironman® in 1986. I was psyched, and ended up doing the Ironman in 1988 (and again in 1995 and 1997). Following Ironman® Europe in 1997, I was pretty burned out on the rigidity and intensity of the triathlon world.

I had seen the Eco-Challenge adventure race on television, and it caught my interest.

Recently forced to retire at the ripe old age of 43, I heard Liz speak one evening in the spring of 1998 at a local outdoor shop in Fort Collins, Colorado, about an adventure race she was helping direct. I didn't really have the skills necessary to complete this 24-hour race—or the guts. Instead I volunteered to house two teams with my family. One of the teams had traveled all the way from New Jersey to Colorado to compete. When that team lost a member due to an emergency the night before the race, I was called into action … and the rest is history.

That race ignited my passion for the outdoors, adventure, and learning new skills. In a very short time, I went from never having touched a climbing harness or kayak paddle in my life to teaching others how to participate in adventure racing at training camps that Liz and I ran. We soon formed MountainQuest Adventures in 1998, a company we designed to provide others with the opportunity to learn about and participate in adventure racing (www.mountain-quest.com).

Together

At about the same time, we both began wondering why most people don't exercise.

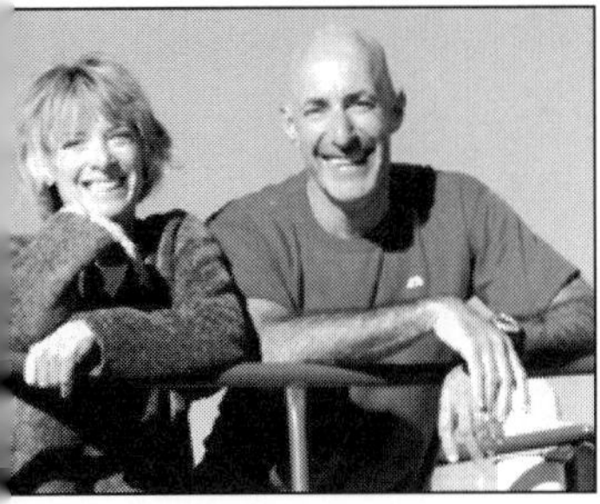

We started asking people that very question. The most frequent answer we received was "because it's not fun." But exercise is fun; maybe it's just people's perception that needs to change. We both know that our perceptions about fitness have changed over the years. Maybe yours can too.

We are not certified personal trainers, nutrition counselors, or physicians. So, rather than give you a scientific formula for fitness we have drawn from our observations and experiences—an approach that we hope you will find to be both refreshing and grounded in reality.

Introduction

Do Americans Need a Department of Exercise?
—Associated Press

Extra Weight Shaves Years Off Lives
—*USA Today*

Fitness: We're in a World of Trouble
—*Omaha World-Herald*

Headlines like these have flooded newspapers, television programs, magazines, and the Internet in recent years, making the topic of health and fitness as commonplace in the media as news items about local school issues and the international economy. These reports tell us that obesity afflicts more than one-third of adults in the United States; that's more than 60 million Americans who are obese, according to the Centers for Disease Control (CDC). Nearly two-thirds of U.S. adults are overweight, or almost 130 million Americans. Being overweight refers to an excess of body weight compared to standards set for muscle, fat, bone, or fluid. Obesity refers specifically to an abnormally high proportion of body fat. Americans' fitness is rapidly deteriorating, and it has become a matter of national concern.

And it should be.

The truth is that we are slowly killing ourselves. People carrying an extra ten to thirty pounds could be shortening their life spans by up to three years. People thirty or more pounds overweight could be losing up to seven years of their lives (Annals of Internal Medicine 138, 2003).

Not only are we killing ourselves, we're also killing our children. For the first time in American history, children are expected to have shorter life spans than their parents, due to obesity-related deaths from illnesses such as heart disease and diabetes, according to the Centers for Disease Control. Some point to television or computer games as the villains.

Others, like us, wonder whether our children's ill health is caused in part by the examples set by their parents and other adults. Federal statistics say that about 60 percent of American adults are not regularly active. About 25 percent are not active *at all* (National Institute of Diabetes and Digestive and Kidney Diseases).

Who can blame them, when the idea of fitness seems expensive, painful, and practically impossible to achieve? It seems that to get on the road to fitness, we need to join a pricey indoor health club and spend hours there. Or, we have to purchase expensive equipment and "nutritional" supplements "guaranteed" to give fast results, or hire a high-priced personal trainer—or all three!

If we get that far, there's not much to look forward to. The word "workout" doesn't suggest joy, or even enjoyment. For most of us, it calls to mind images of men and women slogging nowhere on the treadmill. For others, the picture includes muscle-bound behemoths grunting and sweating while they heave weights around. Most of us watch the clock so we know the second we've done the minimum amount of "exercise" required and can step off the treadmill. How can the idea of fitness possibly entice with mottos like "Feel the Burn" (Jane Fonda's 1980s mantra) or "No Pain, No Gain"? How fun does a get-in-shape "boot camp" sound?

Even if we do manage to "work out," our efforts never seem good enough. Super-thin models on magazine covers and buff exercise gurus hawking their latest home-video, embody an "ideal" weight-level that seems practically impossible for the rest of us to achieve.

We've been intimidated by the media's buff, macho, and unrealistic images, and we've been brainwashed by the commercialized gym mentality. These images and mind-sets appeal to some people. But for most of us, they don't. No wonder so many Americans remain unfit.

The good news is that fitness does not have to be that way. Our goal is to change your ideas about fitness, and give you a new model that redefines "exercise" as simply leading an active, fun lifestyle with plenty of variety.

It's time to get outside and remember the fun we had as kids, when being fit and feeling good were natural outcomes of our active lives. If you're like us, you created games that kept you moving—kickball, hide-and-seek, tag—all while having so much fun that we dreaded being called in for dinner. "Just five more minutes, *please?*" we begged. We're calling for you to simply create a lifestyle defined not by rules and schedules but by enjoyment and diverse activity. We believe the words "fit" and "fun" naturally go together.

During our six-year career as full-time adventure racers, we've talked with athletes, would-be athletes, and non-athletes around the country about endurance and multisport

The goal is to be like the dog that, when he sees his owner open the door, goes crazy and can't wait to get outside to play.

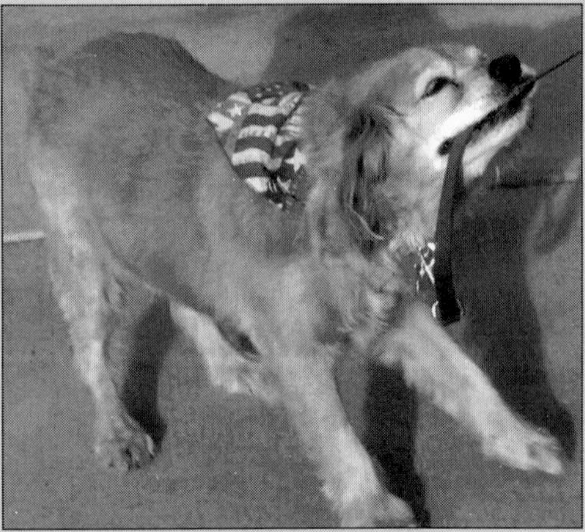

activities. We've met people everywhere with a common goal: to be fit and active. They also want fitness to be fun. In fact, that is why many people take up triathlons or adventure racing: to add variety to their routine, rather than just do the same old (sometimes boring!) thing each day. In other words, mixing activities keeps fitness interesting and fun.

In the pages ahead, we will help you improve your physical and mental well-being by incorporating a fit-and-fun mindset into your life and re-defining yourself as an active person—and you'll get there via a realistic, enjoyable route. We'll start in Chapter 1 by taking stock of our fitness levels. In Chapter 2, we'll talk about a variety of ways to increase those levels. We've dedicated Chapter 3 to exploring the three building blocks of fitness: endurance, strength, and flexibility. In Chapter 4, we'll wrap up with ideas on how to make healthy food choices.

Who knows? Maybe those games of tag and kickball will make you late for dinner again!

CHAPTER 1

Defining Fitness

What does it mean to be "fit"? Having the same size waistline as you had in high school? Being able to run a 10K? One thing is for sure, fitness means more than just an attractive appearance or impressive physical strength. To some degree, those are natural outcomes of being fit. But they are not the main goal.

To us, being fit means being healthy—that is, staying free of illness, being active, and feeling good about yourself.

A fit person is like a tuned car. Whereas the untuned car chugs along but occasionally stalls or breaks down, a tuned car runs smoothly and with maximum fuel efficiency. When we are fit, our heart, lungs, blood vessels, and muscles

Good (and Fit) Old Abe

***Abe Kukawka** was born in 1910. At age 65, he began walking and he still walks every day. In fact, at age 93, he continues to rise at 5 a.m., looking forward to seeing his friends at the Jewish Community Center in Omaha, Nebraska, and to walking his daily three miles. "I go up on the roof and I clean my gutters; I do all of my own yard work, and I shovel the snow," Abe says. "If I couldn't do all of these things, I'd sell the house." Being active is an essential part of Abe's life. It's something he enjoys and is proud of.*

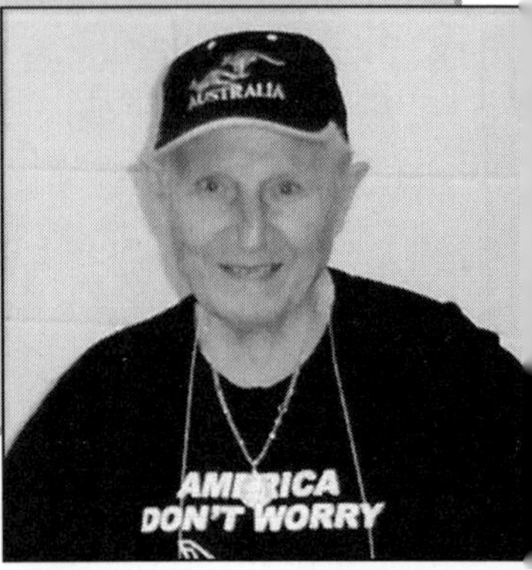

perform optimally. The benefits of fitness are well documented—increased energy, protection from certain diseases, and a greater sense of well-being.

What do we mean by "active"? Federal guidelines define it as thirty minutes or more of activity every day. The National Academies' Institute of Medicine recommends an hour of moderate activity daily for weight control and health benefits. As for us, we say just get out there and move around … pretty regularly.

Part of the problem is that technology has made it so easy for us to avoid activity. You can buy anything you want via the Internet without even leaving your home. Food, ready to eat, can be delivered right to your door. Don't rake the leaves, the television commercials tell us; buy a leaf blower! Television and other media magnets draw us in twenty-four hours a day, seven days a week. As technology has become more pervasive in our society, we've lost opportunities in our daily lives to stay active and maintain a naturally healthy lifestyle.

So, with those ideas in mind, we want you to become more conscious of being active. Period. It's definitely smart to start with small steps, in which you would first make an effort to be active in some way for, let's say, thirty minutes per day three to five days a week. That would be a great starting point. If you gradually increased the duration to forty-five minutes or more four or five days a week, you would certainly begin to qualify as leading an active lifestyle.

Does Thin Equal Fit?

The size of a person's body does not necessarily indicate their level of health or fitness, as Covert Bailey pointed out in 1978 in his book *Fit or Fat.* Before then, the picture of ideal male fitness meant lots of muscles à la Arnold Schwarzenegger. All you need to do is watch a popular television show to see that the model of fitness for women has become progressively skinnier over the years.

However, thin people may be carrying an unhealthy percentage of fat. How can that be? Let's think back to when we were active kids and burned calories as fast as we ate them. As adults, unfortunately, things changed, and we became less active. As a result, our muscles started to become less lean and more fatty. It is important to realize that during this process, our weight may not have changed. We may proudly tell everyone that we still weigh the same as we did in high school. This is an accomplishment, but it doesn't mean you've maintained the same amount of muscle. Fat may simply be replacing the unused muscle. It's only when the fat begins to deposit outside the muscle sheath, because it has run out of room, that we notice the accumulation of fat and its accompanying weight gain.

Individuals of every size need activity, to kick-start their metabolism and turn calories and fat into healthier muscle.

Mind, Body, and Spirit

Fitness isn't just about physical activity. It includes the emotional stability and mental ability that come from maintaining a certain level of physical activity, decent nutrition, and accepting who you are. We should quit thinking about being "in shape," and assess our level of fitness in terms of both physical and emotional health.

A large part of feeling fit and being healthy relates to how we view ourselves. Creating a more positive outlook will bring us closer to our goal of being fit. Abe Kukawka, a 93-year-old man from Omaha, is a fit individual. His daily activity keeps him not only physically active, but also mentally positive. You may never look like a super model, but you can

The Complete Connection

***Marialice Wilson** and **Calvin Wetzel** wake up every morning raring to go. They don't have to, now that they are both retired, but they can't wait to get the day started. "This renewed vigor," Marialice says, "we owe, in part, to the ancient practice of Tai Chi." While they both talk happily about the physical benefit to their strength and flexibility (Marialice is a half inch taller than she used to be!), it is the sense of well-being and calmness that they get from regular Tai Chi practice that keep them at it.*

Tai Chi does not require any equipment, so the couple is able to do it even when they travel. They have practiced Tai Chi on the rim of the Grand Canyon, among the ruins at Wupatki National Monument in Arizona, and on the beaches of the North Carolina coast.

continued on page 16

continued from page 15

"We experience a sense of connection with the earth, and a serenity, while practicing Tai Chi—especially when we practice outdoors," Marialice and Calvin say. They understand and embrace the mind-body-spirit connection and are busy teaching others how to practice the gentle art of Tai Chi, and incorporate it into their lives to feel better, improve health, and eliminate stress.

For more information on Tai Chi, visit ***www.taoist.org***.

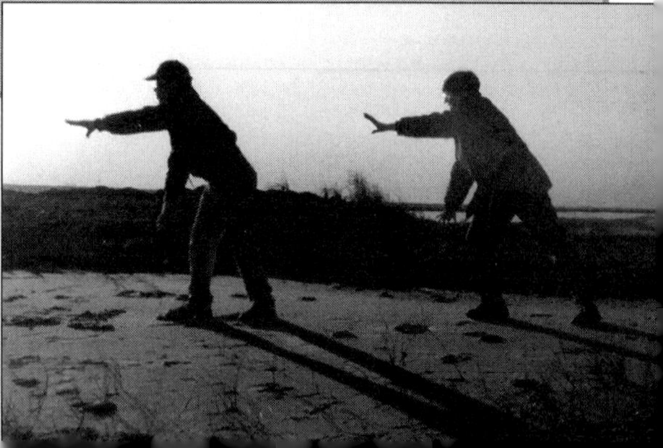

attain fitness and health and celebrate that accomplishment. A positive state of mind is a wonderful by-product of being fit!

Assessing Your Level of Fitness

So, how do you get started on the road to total fitness? The first step is to be honest about your current levels of strength, endurance, and flexibility.

Throw away the scale … for now. Body *weight* may not tell you what you really need to know about your level of fitness. Body *composition* gives a more accurate picture of health, because it shows what percentage of our weight comes from dense matter such as bone, muscle, body organs, as well as fat. One way of assessing your body composition is by estimating your body mass index (BMI). You can calculate your BMI by consulting health and fitness Web sites such as **www.ivillage.com**.

A BMI of 18.5 to 24.9 is considered normal, with no associated increase in health risk. A BMI of 25 to 29.9 is considered overweight and over 30 is classified as obese (NIH, 1998).

Another measure of health is your body fat percentage. A healthy percentage for women is 13 to 25 percent of total body weight. For men, the range is 8 to 20 percent. A body fat percentage of more than 32 percent of body weight for women, and 25 percent for men, is considered obese.

While we're on the subject of fat, remember that fat isn't necessarily bad. We all need some for the healthy maintenance of our internal organs. But in excess, there's no doubt … it is bad. Don't feel that you have to know your body fat composition before increasing your level of activity. Suffice it to say, you want to keep your body fat "low," not "high."

Besides taking a look at your body composition and body fat, you can also evaluate your physical fitness in terms of three key areas: muscle strength, endurance, and flexibility. The following are some simple ways to look at your current fitness level in each of these areas. Our goal here is not to discourage you and make you wake up early every morning to do push-ups, sit-ups, and pull-ups. We simply want you to understand some of the components of a fully fit body and, perhaps, encourage activity to improve some of these key areas.

The easiest way to measure abdominal strength (sometimes called "core" strength) is to do sit-ups or crunches. For upper-body strength, do push-ups. Running is a good indicator of your endurance level. Then we'll show you some ways to assess your flexibility and range of motion.

Core Strength: Crunches

Crunches (or sit-ups) strengthen the underlying muscles within your abdominal area. The basic technique is to lie on the floor with your feet hip-width apart and your knees bent. Cross your arms across your chest with your hands resting just below your shoulders (or, hands behind your head and neck). While keeping your head absolutely straight and looking upward, raise your shoulders off the ground several inches. You should feel your abdominal muscles contract. Hold for a moment, and release back to the starting position.

Crunch Averages for Men

Age	<35	36–45	45+
Excellent	60	50	40
Good	45	40	25
Fair	30	25	15

Crunch Averages for Women

Age	<35	36–45	45+
Excellent	50	40	30
Good	40	25	15
Fair	25	15	10

For beginners, count the number of crunches you can do without pausing. Compare your results to our table. A more advanced test involves holding a dumbbell (with both hands) on your chest, while doing this exercise. The dumbbell should equal 10 to 20 percent of your body weight. More than ten crunches is excellent.

Upper-Body Strength: Push-Ups

Push-ups are the easiest and best way to assess and build upper-body strength. The correct technique for a push-up is to lie on the floor facing down, your legs out straight, toes on the floor, and your feet eight to twelve inches apart. Place your hands on the floor, a couple of inches outside your shoulders, with your fingers pointing forward. Keeping your back as straight as possible (head, neck, and spine all aligned), and your abdominal muscles tight, raise your body up and slowly lower yourself to the floor until your chest lightly touches the floor. Repeat. Women may choose to modify this position by keeping their knees bent on the floor. Do not arch your back or look up.

For beginners, count the number of push-ups you can do slowly and deliberately without stopping, and compare to our table. Our advanced test has you place your feet on a stability ball or a chair, with your hands on the

Push-up Averages for Men

Age	20–29	30–39	40–49	50–59	60+
Excellent	45+	35+	30+	25+	20+
Good	35–44	25–34	20–29	15–24	10–19
Fair	20–34	15–24	12–19	8–14	5–9

Push-up Averages for Women

Age	20–29	30–39	40–49	50–59	60+
Excellent	34+	25+	20+	15+	5+
Good	17–33	12–24	8–19	6–14	3–4
Fair	6–16	4–11	3–7	2–5	1–2

floor, and do as many decline position push-ups as you can without stopping. More than ten decline push-ups for women, and twenty for men, is excellent.

Cardiovascular Endurance: Running

Run or walk briskly for half a mile and record your time. If you cover the distance in less than ten minutes walking or less than six minutes running, you are on the way to building an excellent endurance base.

Flexibility: Range of Motion

Flexibility and range of motion allow you to maintain your endurance and strength through the years. We're 49 in 2004 and still going strong!

Warm up with a short walk or jog before doing these tests. Bend at the waist and reach for the floor. If you can easily touch the floor, your flexibility is good. Our advanced test, which tests the flexibility in your shoulders, has you stand up and raise your right arm. Bend your arm at the elbow. At the same time, reach your left arm around your back. See if you can make your right and left hands touch. Now switch, and try the opposite arms. If you can clasp your hands behind your back, your flexibility in this area is excellent.

Once you know your fitness level in each of these areas, you can set a course for future goals. It's really important at this stage to acknowledge your fitness level without judgment. This is not the time to beat yourself up. Instead, focus on the fact that you have decided to take steps to improve your fitness and health. Establishing that positive mindset is a great place to start your journey toward fitness and fun.

CHAPTER 2

Taking That First Step

We surveyed people from a variety of backgrounds about fitness. Overwhelmingly, the biggest obstacle to fitness is the inability to "stick with it." Every January people sign up with a health club with the best intentions of getting fit. Three months later, the health clubs are empty and the majority of people have given up. Less than 20 percent of the U.S. population is considered fit, and 61 percent of American adults are overweight, according to the Federal Trade Commission. Millions of people don't make the effort to stay healthy.

Why is that? Here's our list of Top Ten Excuses for Why People Are Not Fit (with a nod to David Letterman).

10. One more donut.
9. I don't belong to a health club.
8. I have two left feet. (I'm uncoordinated.)
7. I live in Alaska.
6. I need a coach/trainer.
5. I don't know how to get started.
4. The couch is too comfortable.
3. I don't have time.
2. I can't afford it.
1. I can't stick with it.

Let's focus on reasons one through three: No time, no money, and it's just too hard.

Being Fit Takes Time (That I Don't Have!)

We are not advocating that you dedicate huge chunks of each day to being active. Rather, focus on incorporating activity into your everyday life. There are 1,440 minutes in each day. Being active for thirty of them is easy! It does take time to be fit—but not as much as you may think. Remember, becoming fit simply means becoming more active. Integrate your activities into your daily life, so that doing them becomes convenient. Find fun ways to get fit and build your endurance without even realizing you are doing it. Pick things you can do any time or any place.

Walking is a great example. We're willing to bet that you can find the time to do a few of these activities:

- Walk during lunch or coffee breaks at work.
- Walk or ride your bike with your kids to their school or daycare.
- Go for a walk with your spouse after dinner. Let the kids do the dishes! Schedule one night a week to walk with each of your kids. Let them talk about anything. You'll be amazed at how fit you both become—physically and emotionally.

For some, making the time means giving something else up (how about one hour of television?), getting up earlier in the morning, or going outside during your lunch break. If, however, you need to "schedule" your new activities, starting out at thirty minutes a day four to five days per week is an excellent way to go.

Multitasking

Bonnie Faranosi *was feeling crunched for time. Not only was she working forty hours per week, but she also was using all her spare time to study for exams to become a board-certified diagnostic medical sonographer. She missed getting outside on the trails near her home in Fort Collins, Colorado, but she was determined to put in the necessary study time. Her solution? She created study note cards and studied while she hiked!*

Being Fit Costs Too Much

Creating a more active lifestyle does not necessarily require a financial investment. For starters, try walking to the store or library. Take the stairs at work rather than the elevator. Think about easy, low- or no-cost ways to incorporate more movement into your daily routine.

Rebecca Rusch knows it's possible. One of the top adventure racers in the world, and one of the fittest women around, Rebecca doesn't belong to a health club. She's got the great outdoors. For about five years, she lived out of her truck, picking up enough work wherever she could to buy food and pay her bills. We're not saying you should leave your home for this lifestyle. The point is that Rebecca's fitness does not depend on her bank account. She skis, runs, bikes, paddles, and climbs—all outdoors, and all while living on a shoestring.

Fit and Fun with Frisbees

Remember Wham-O, the company that brought us the Frisbee in 1958? The plastic disc has spawned a couple of full-fledged sports that offer unique and fun fitness opportunities. Ultimate Frisbee, for example, involves aspects of football, soccer, field hockey, and lots of fun in a team-sport setting. See **www.upa.org** *for more information.*

In Disc Golf, an activity started in the 1970s, a Frisbee takes the place of both the golf ball and clubs. Players throw discs into a specially designed basket, or hole. The Professional Disc Golf Association boasts over 24,000 members, and disc-golf courses have sprung up all around the country. Check it out at

***www.pdga.com**. Or how about just getting out there with your dog and having a blast throwing the Frisbee for him. Your dog will love it and, again, you'll be having fun while being active outdoors.*

No dog? Well, it's still fun to play the original game of Frisbee catch with a partner. You see, being active does not have to be traditional or cost a lot of money. You can buy a Frisbee for about $5.

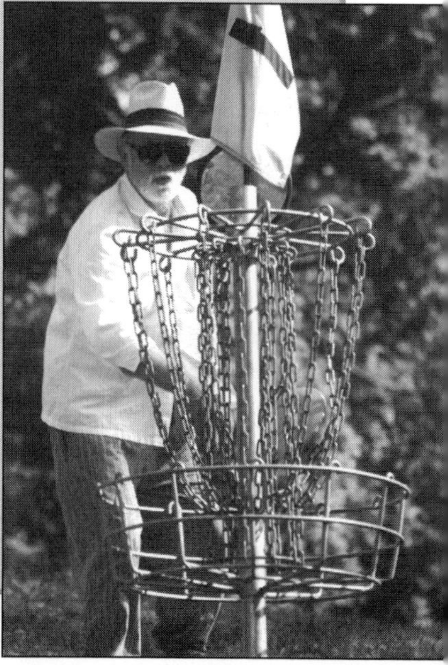

Getting Fit Is Just Not Fun!

Let's face it, the idea of getting fit simply doesn't inspire most Americans. For example, let's take a look at the terms typically used to describe how to get fit—especially "working out" and "exercising." How many people, after a hard day at work, feel like "working (out)" even more, particularly when their busy schedules afford little room for it? Even the idea of "exercising" sounds exhausting, like a chore we've got to finish.

We think it's time to change our ideas about how to get fit.

We propose striking terminology like "working out" and "exercise" from your vocabulary. Instead, let's start talking about getting outside, being active, and having fun. Getting fit can be fun—if you approach it with a joyful attitude. We are going to help you begin to redefine yourself as an active person, with an active lifestyle. In a shorter time than you would imagine possible, an increase in activity will put you on the road to fitness and better health. The key is to make your activity fun. It should not, and doesn't have to, feel like work or something you have to do. We're going to help you look for ways to be active that you'll want to do, simply because you enjoy them.

Cruising for Fun

So, you don't have a fancy bike, or aren't comfortable wearing those tight Lycra cycling shorts? No worries. There is a new—or, rather, old—cycling movement in action: the return of the ***cruiser bike.*** *Ski towns such as Aspen and Crested Butte in Colorado are famous for their "townie" bikes, and those old fat tire, high handlebar, single-speed bikes are now being seen more and more frequently everywhere. In fact, the Thursday Evening Cruiser Rides in Boulder, Colorado, routinely attract 100*

continued on page 34

continued from page 33

to 200 riders who are out for a fun, leisurely jaunt through town. Find a single speed or other older or inexpensive bike from a thrift store or a recycled sporting goods retailer and get out there in a fun, non-competitive way. You should see the smiles you get when you cruise around town, and you know what? Those smiles are very contagious.

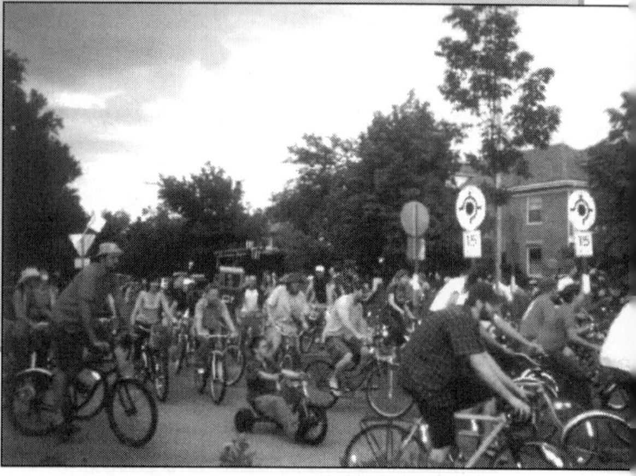

Your daily fitness must hold your interest without being punishing. Try to pick something you will look forward to and will enjoy doing. Maybe it's a morning walk (with that cup of coffee in hand), taking a yoga class, riding that old bike of yours around the neighborhood, or playing Frisbee with your child, spouse, or dog in a large field.

How about making your activities social? Invite a friend to come with you on a regular basis. You're more likely to go if you've committed to someone else, and almost any activity is more fun with a friend along. Join a group, such as a hiking or biking club and make new, active friends. Or, try a new activity. How about bike polo, volleyball, or inline skating?

Whatever activity you choose, two rules apply. Rule 1: Make sure it's fun. Rule 2: Just do it!

Pair Power

Doing anything is more fun when you share it with a friend—and that's especially true when you can accomplish a fitness or health goal together. Let others know what your goals are. You'll be pleasantly surprised to find others with a similar goal. There is power in support and you might even make a new friend or two along the way.

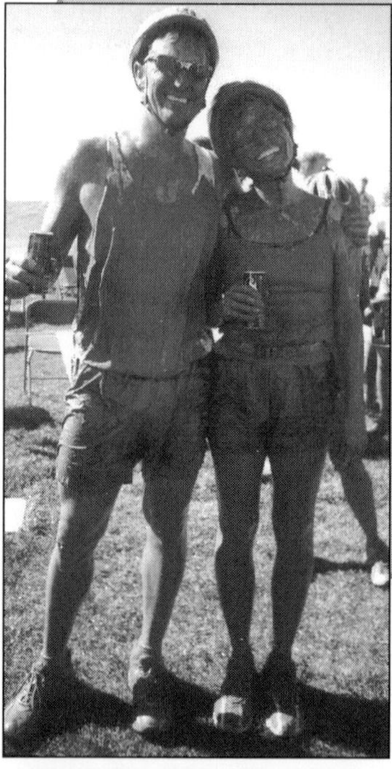

Go Fly a Kite

*Fly a kite? Why not! If the standard old string and $2.99 Superman kite at Wal-Mart doesn't excite you, how about kite sailing or kite skiing? **Jason Middleton** used his kite flying and aeronautical skills to speed up his boat at Eco-Challenge Borneo in 2000, a maneuver that propelled his team to first place early in the race! You can also try kite surfing, kite mountain boarding, stunt kiting. Or, try kite skating ... on inline skates. Why not have some fun getting out there by starting with Superman? Then maybe think of something crazy!*

Other potential obstacles to daily activity include uncooperative weather, travel, and family obligations. There's not much you can do to change the weather, but you can plan for it. Make sure you have appropriate clothing for the weather. Or have back-up plans. For example, if it's raining, take a brisk walk in the local mall. You can also use the "bad" weather to your advantage. Grab an umbrella and go stomp in a few puddles!

If you are on the road on a business trip, take a jump rope with you. Or take a walk to scout out your new surroundings. We travel all around the world and have found that one of the best things to do in a new place is to immediately get outside for a walk or run. Our motive isn't always fitness. It gives us a chance to read the menus posted in the restaurant windows so we can pick the most interesting place to eat!

Family Time

*For **Todd Fields,** the fun started when his son got fed up with baseball and looked for a new sport to play. He decided on lacrosse. But when Todd discovered that the community had no team, he suddenly found himself starting a lacrosse league for kids in his community. He learned everything he could about the sport and coached and practiced with the kids. A runner most of his adult life, he joined a masters lacrosse league in Denver. At the age of 41, he learned to play a team sport for the first time. "I've never had so much fun in my life," he says. "I admit that half the fun is telling war stories after the game. But the best part is that lacrosse is a game I can play with my kids."*

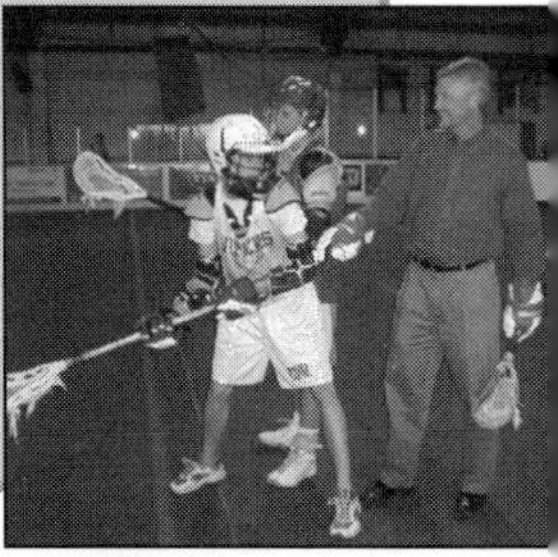

People with families can be active, too. Take your children with you in a stroller or backpack, or let them hike along. Some kids might even want to bike or skate while you walk or jog. When Barry started training for his first marathon in 1981, his 2-year-old son and wife went on every run with him, on a bike. Brian sat happily in his mom's bike-carrier seat while holding his dad's water bottle.

Set Goals

Why do people give up their efforts at getting fit? They often set unrealistic goals. They try to undo the damage from years of poor eating habits and lack of exercise by working out like crazy, and end up with injuries, sore muscles, and defeated ambitions.

Setting realistic goals is an important key to the success of a lifestyle fitness program. First, identify what is most important to you. Do you want to lose weight or lower your cholesterol and triglyceride levels? Is reducing your body fat percentage most important? Do you want to run a 5K road race or a triathlon, or have more defined abdominal muscles? Make sure that you select reasonable and healthy goals by keeping your current fitness level in mind. It's always best to consult with your physician, fitness expert, or nutritionist about your goals. Here are some examples of long-term goals:

- Reduce jeans size from 14 to 10.
- Hike the Grand Canyon.
- Do a triathlon.
- Lower percentage of body fat. (Ask your doctor to check your current level and help you set a reasonable goal.)

After you've identified a big-picture goal, select two or three small, recognizable and specific short-term goals to achieve along the way. These "stepping stones" will motivate you to stay on the program. These are some examples of short-term goals:

- Be able to walk or run for twenty minutes without stopping.
- Walk to the grocery store one day per week.
- Do eight push-ups and twenty sit-ups without stopping.

Write down your goals and put them in a prominent place, such as on the refrigerator door, to remind you of your dream. Research indicates that people who write down their goals tend to achieve them in the long run. Gary Scott, an international mountain guide, author of *Summit Strategies* (2003), and simply a great guy, suggests that when you set a long-term goal (climbing Everest, in his case) schedule it on a particular date. Write it on the calendar. Tell your boss and friends, and start working toward it.

Tennis to Marathoning 101

In 1981, ***Barry*** *was getting burned out on playing tennis in Detroit's competitive clubs. Then he read that the* Detroit Free Press *newspaper sponsored a major international marathon each year. The paper also printed a daily training schedule. If readers were able to run or jog five miles initially, and if they followed the schedule, they would reach the marathon finish line in just three months! After following the training schedule strictly for three months, Barry finished his first marathon in three hours, fifty-nine minutes. That was just the start of his endurance sporting life. (To learn more, see "Barry's Story" in the Preface.)*

If you can find a path with no obstacles, it probably doesn't lead anywhere.

—Anonymous

You gain strength, courage, and confidence by every experience in which you stop to look fear in the face. You must do the thing which you think you cannot do.

—Eleanor Roosevelt

Another effective approach is to keep building on your short-term goals. For example, after you have successfully reached your goal number of push-ups and sit-ups, up the ante and set a new goal. For example, try adding pull-ups or increasing the number of days you do them per week. Setting new goals not only helps you track your progress, but it also keeps your activities interesting and keeps you motivated.

Toy Soldiers Go Step by Step

In 1997, four friends in New Jersey were watching television and saw a broadcast of the ***Eco-Challenge Race,*** *the granddaddy of all multiday, multisport adventure races. They immediately decided that they had to do it themselves! They formed a team, called it Toy Soldiers, and started doing short three to four-hour adventure races on the East Coast. They even set up a Web site and boldly stated their goal of competing in the Eco-Challenge. Well, it took five years and dozens of races. But in 2001, Team Toy Soldiers proudly competed in—and finished—the Eco-Challenge in New Zealand. They set a long-term goal, and their short-term goals helped them achieve it.*

It is important to maintain the new level of activity of the short-term goal for a period before moving on to the next goal. If, for example, you wanted to do two more push-ups every other day, be sure you have done this for a week or two, until it has become a normal and comfortable part of your lifestyle. Then try adding something new.

Reward yourself when you have achieved each of your short-term goals. Food doesn't always have to be the reward, although a peppermint patty can be a nice treat. Maybe you can use clothes, shoes, or music as occasional rewards. Celebrate the fact that you're on your way to making fitness a part of your life!

CHAPTER 3

Fitness Fundamentals

You've given your fitness level a reality check and admitted that you'd like to be more active. You've even set some initial short-term and long-term goals. Now let's get started on your fitness quest. Remember to make it a time of joy, not obligation, by engaging your mind and spirit as well as your body.

Let's start by focusing on the three fundamental elements of fitness: endurance, strength, and flexibility. All three can help you achieve an ideal level of fitness. You don't need to stress about which one to do first, because most activities will naturally include aspects of all three elements, although some do emphasize one or two elements more than others.

How do these elements contribute to fitness? *Endurance* is another way of talking about the heart's capacity, or ability, to do aerobic work. It allows you to climb the hill to watch a sunset. *Strength* helps to prevent injury, improve balance, and protect your bones as you age. *Flexibility* is often an overlooked element of fitness. But, without it, our endurance and strength can only go so far. We often hear people in their fifties and older say, "I'd (run, swim, bike) but my (knees, back, legs) hurt when I do anything like that." Working on flexibility prevents many of those aches and pains and helps to balance muscles and maintain core strength. It's never too late to start to improve flexibility.

All three components of fitness contribute to healthy bones and muscles and help to prevent diseases. Getting fit isn't just about sweating and burning calories—the holy

No One's Perfect

*We, **Liz** and **Barry,** know we should include some concentration on flexibility in our playtime—especially as we get older. But admittedly it's the last thing either of us makes an effort to include. We'll have to work on that one with you!*

grail of the seventies, eighties, and nineties. Today's approach might be more beneficial, because it creates a strong, healthy body, while cultivating a peaceful frame of mind. For example, martial arts and yoga blend physical, mental, and spiritual traditions and build endurance, strength, and flexibility while focusing on breathing and the mind-body union. Mindfully incorporate endurance, strength, and flexibility into your life.

Trade in Your Horses

Bike polo? *Believe it or not this sport is thought to have evolved over a century ago in India when British soldiers were looking for a way to maintain their polo skills. Today bike polo is played all over the world. The obvious advantage — you can have all of the fun and challenge without the high cost. All you need is a bicycle, helmet, short mallet, and a bicycle polo ball. You can play on any level playing field, but preferably on grass since falls happen! Each team has four players and the standard polo rules apply.*

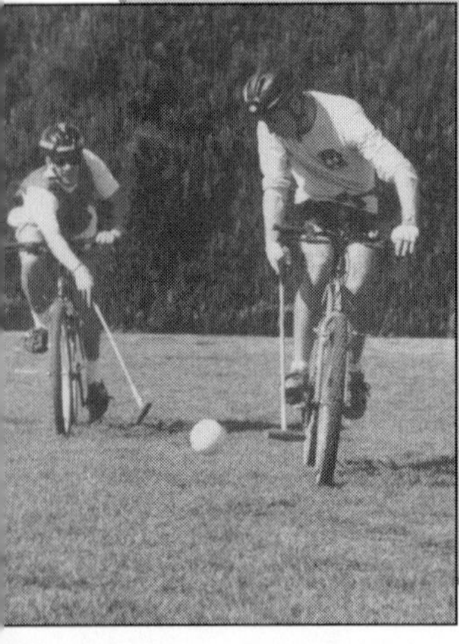

www.bikepolo.com

Top Ten Reasons Bike Polo is Better than Mountain or Road Biking

10. *It's hard to go mountain biking without mountains, but almost everyone has a soccer field nearby.*
9. *There's no need to carry your water—you're never more than 100 yards from a cooler.*
8. *There's no need to carry tools or spare bike parts.*
7. *Fancy suspension on your bike is unnecessary.*
6. *There's no need for more than one gear.*
5. *When you fall it's usually on soft grass at a slow speed.*
4. *You'll never have to carry your bike more than 100 yards—even if it breaks.*
3. *You probably won't be hit by a car.*
2. *Hitting the ball is a great way to take out some aggression.*
1. *You get to play a game, not just go for a ride.*

Building Endurance

Endurance is simply your body's ability to function aerobically (which means you can breathe!) for a sustained period. Endurance means your ability to hike, walk around the block, swim, and play tag. In short, endurance makes it possible to enjoy life. To build endurance, you need to engage in steady, sustained activity of moderate intensity. In plain English, that means you need to get off your butt and do something active—anything—for a continuous period. Almost any activity that increases your breathing and heart rate will build endurance.

And speaking of the heart, as you slowly build your capacity to keep active for longer periods, you are strengthening your heart. After a while, you may even notice your resting pulse rate (the number of beats your heart makes per minute) going down. The lower your resting pulse, the less your heart has to work and—all things being equal—the longer it will last!

Boot-Scootin' Works up a Sweat

***William "Bubba" Jones** lost weight equivalent to a whole person—200 pounds! How'd he do it? Not by going to the gym every day. Surprised? Instead, he went dancing ... line dancing, to be exact. Now he teaches line dancing to enthusiastic learners of all ages in Knoxville, Tennessee. People stomp, strut, twirl, and slide across the floor, all while laughing and sweating.* (Knoxville News Sentinel, *Aug. 2003)*

When Kenneth H. Cooper first proposed the concept of aerobics in 1968, he advocated intense periods of exercise—and the more the better. Today, he and some of his colleagues at the Cooper Institute for Aerobics Research in Dallas have scaled back their recommendations, saying that running fifteen miles a week is all you need to maintain fitness. Not all of

Kenneth's colleagues agree, saying that increasing the challenge as you become more fit is still a good way to go. Either way, most fitness experts agree that to build endurance you need to engage in thirty minutes of aerobic activity three to four times per week.

Walk This Way

Since 1979, members of the ***American Volksport Association*** *from around the country have trekked many thousands of miles in U.S. cities, towns, parks, forests, rural areas—anywhere they've found a pleasant or interesting place to walk. The Volkssport Association, an international walking group dedicated to exercising for fun, fellowship, and fitness, charts year-round walking trails and stages annual walking events. Members walk trails that*

But that doesn't mean you have to do thirty minutes all at once. Get outside and do it in increments, if you like. For example, take ten minutes to briskly walk the dog in the morning before work, and then do twenty minutes of biking or inline skating with your children after work.

they had driven past for years and didn't even know existed. They set goals, like walking charted trails in every state, or walking Route 66. "When you see it on foot, you really see the city or the countryside," members say.

Many states have Volkssport chapters. The association's book, The Starting Point *(updated yearly), describes more than 1,000 self-guided walks throughout the United States. Get more information online at* ***www.ava.org****.*

Studies show just getting off the couch and doing anything aerobic has the greatest health benefit. Beyond that, increasing your athletic level only produces a small health benefit. So don't worry about the intensity or time involved—just get moving.

Your only concern is to start, get out, and enjoy it. Do it without any expectations or rules. Leave your watch at home and stay out as long as you're having fun. There are many exciting and fun ways to incorporate building endurance into your daily life. The key is to choose activities you enjoy. The main point is to start. Sometimes just getting out the door can be the hardest part. Here are a few ideas of activities you may want to begin:

- wash your car
- play volleyball
- garden
- walk

Get High

... on a flying trapeze, that is. Even if you don't plan on joining the circus, a trapeze session can improve your balance, timing, strength, body awareness, and your belief in your ability to do more than you imagined you could. And we haven't even talked about the adrenaline rush of jumping off the platform. At Trapeze School New York in New York City, the motto is "Forget fear. Worry about the addiction."

- walk the stairs at work
- shovel snow
- jump on a trampoline
- ride a bike
- skate—ice, roller, or inline

For more ideas, log on to **www.presidents challenge.org**.

Developing Strength

Strength refers to more than beefy arm muscles. When we refer to strength, we usually mean *core strength,* or your midsection's capacity for exertion. The body's core includes the muscles of the lower back, abdomen, and buttocks. You use core strength in almost all movements and activities. Before anything in your body can move, the midsection must move first. A solid core transfers power from the lower body to the upper body—like when you lift those grocery bags or a child, or put a backpack on your back.

Building strength can improve endurance as well as provide these benefits:

- maintain balance
- prevent injuries
- increase speed and power
- ease work for your heart and lungs
- balance musculature and strengthen your body's core

Skijoring

If you own a big, healthy dog and a pair of cross-country skis, why stay indoors this winter? You could start practicing for the next potential winter Olympic sport: ***skijoring.*** *A Norwegian word meaning "ski-driving," skijoring involves a cross-country skier using a dog (or dogs) to pull them across the snow. Sorry, you're not just along for the ride. It does take skill and effort. All you need is a willing dog, a dog harness, skis, a bungee-type cord, and a waist harness or climbing harness to connect you to the dog. It's a great way to spend time with the pooch. No snow? No worries. Try bike-joring instead!* ***www.skijornow.com.***

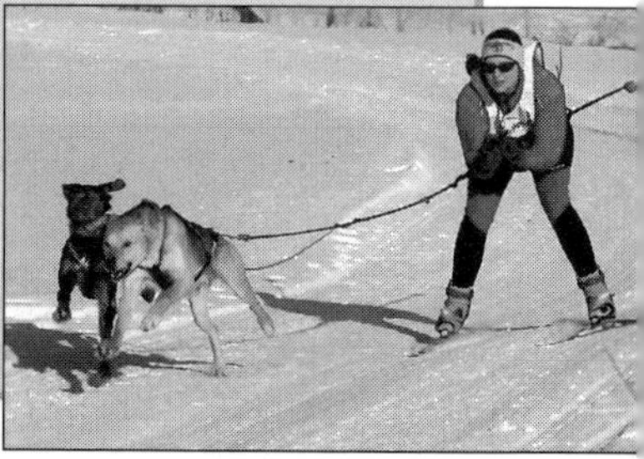

- make your body leaner
- decrease bone loss

Many strength-building programs require the equipment normally found in an indoor gym. But there are other ways to build strength outdoors. Here are some examples:

- stepping up (use a picnic-table bench or low retaining wall)
- monkey bars (great for pull-ups or just cross rung by rung from one end to the other)
- arm dips (use low retaining walls or benches)
- bound or skip uphill
- walking lunges for the length of a field or your sidewalk

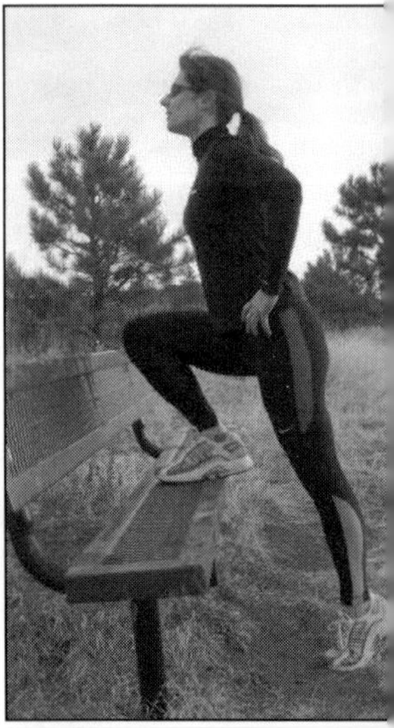

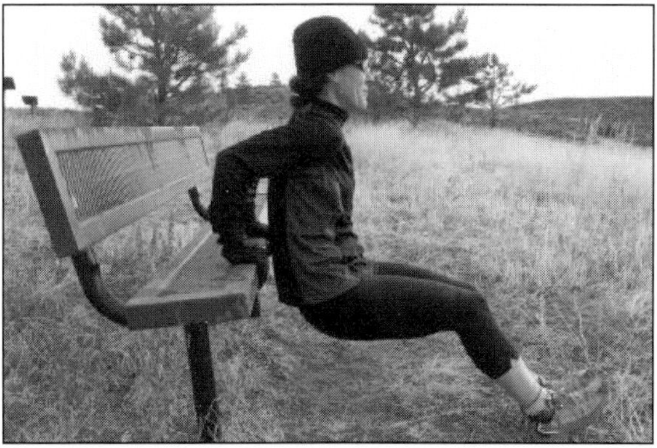

Becoming Flexible

Over time, daily activities tighten our muscles. Running, for example, can create inflexible hamstring muscles. Mountain biking tends to constrict the hip flexors. Aging can also tighten our muscles, so that taking those first steps out of bed in the morning gets harder. To reverse that natural tendency, it's important to stretch and elongate the muscles. Be sure to warm up the body before stretching. A good time to stretch is after being active and playing. Here are six core muscle groups you can focus on:

- hamstrings
- quadriceps
- calves and Achilles tendons
- shoulders
- back

A popular method for improving flexibility, while building strength, is yoga. This ancient meditative technique involves a series of poses that tone and stretch the body and help make you aware of your breathing. Some of the benefits of yoga include:

- enhanced muscle tone
- improved balance
- increased flexibility, strength, and endurance
- improved breathing technique
- improved concentration

Top athletes from a variety of sports, like Florida Marlins pitcher Carl Pavano, find that yoga gives them a competitive edge in their sport and prevents injury. The benefits of mental focus and concentration, as well as physical strength flexibility, are worth any flack he gets from his less "enlightened" teammates.

Here are some basic poses you may want to try:

- Sun Salutation
- Warrior
- Triangle
- Tree
- Downward Dog

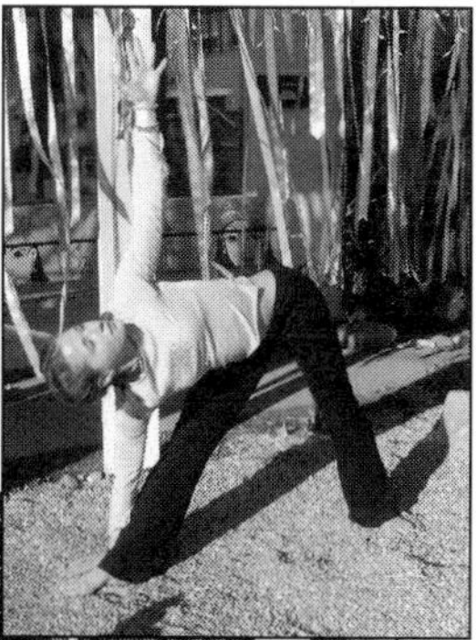

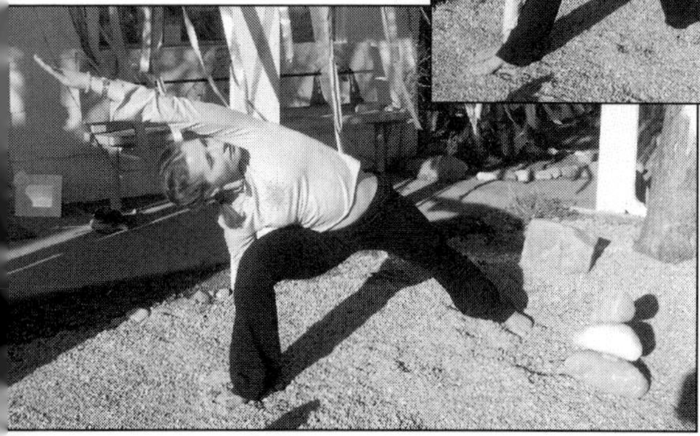

Like flexibility, good balance and agility also contribute to fitness. Whether you are hiking, biking, climbing, or doing any other active movement, being agile will help you do it better and easier. A fun way to improve your agility is by putting yourself in safe, unbalanced situations. How about learning to skateboard or inline skate? Play flashlight tag at night with the kids, or walk on rocks in a river, which we do to practice for our adventure races. Walk on a curb or across a log to improve your balance. The point is, have fun!

Paying attention to the fitness triad of endurance, strength, and flexibility will not only make you a more rounded fitness "*fun*damentalist" but will also offer you an almost endless choice of activities.

Footbagging

When is the last time you did a toe-reverse, slap down, or scuff? No, they're not boxing moves. They're part of a standard Footbag competition. Remember the old hacky-sack days, when those laid-back groups of kids stood in a circle kicking around a little sand-filled bag? Well, the sport has grown up. Now you'll find exciting competitions

continued on page 66

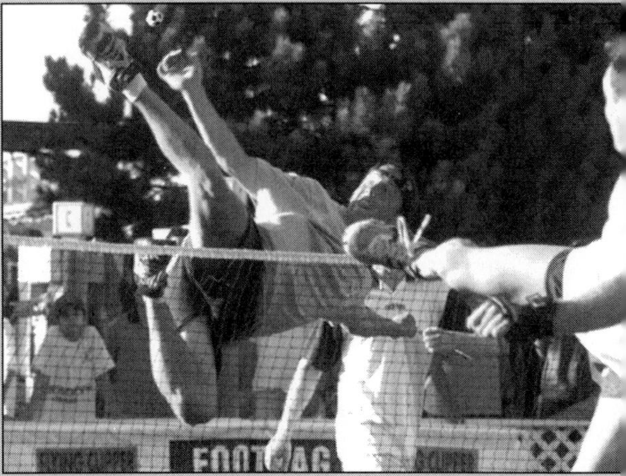

continued from page 65

everywhere in the world, and even a hotly contested world championship competition. The event includes Freestyle Footbagging, which requires tremendous athletic ability likened by competitors to the demands of gymnastics. Athletes jump, hop, and use balance to perform stunts. Then there's Footbag Net, an intense team sport similar to beach volleyball, played on a court with a five-foot high net! Footbagging can be done by any one, any time. All you need is a footbag. "It can add hours of fun to each day," says **Chris Ott,** *national marketing director of the International Footbag Players Association. "A footbag easily fits into a pocket or purse so you can take it everywhere. You'll be amazed at how quickly you improve your flexibility, balance, and strength!"* ***www.footbag.org***

CHAPTER 4

Eating Consciously

We often tell people that if we weren't active, we'd be fighting a major battle against midlife bulge. You see, both of us love to eat. We love good, nutritious food, but we also love our own indulgences. For us, that means sweets. Barry usually has a giant bag of Mike and Ikes chewy candies nearby, and Liz can tell you where to find the best cinnamon roll anywhere in the country. We know we shouldn't eat this way all the time—but, hey, we're human too, so we factor the occasional treat into our lifestyle. We can get away with it mostly because we're so active.

So we won't tell you to abstain from all the foods you love. We won't even try to convince you that you'll soon like the taste of nutritiously prepared food and will never crave anything salty, greasy, or sweet again. Instead we'll share some ideas to help you become aware of what you eat and learn to emphasize the good stuff and minimize the not-so-good stuff. We think that's a reasonable way to keep eating simple, healthy, and interesting.

The Junk-Food Habit

For most of us, life is fast and full of conveniences. That includes the way we approach food, too. Most people don't cook or eat at home as much as the generations that came before us. Thirty percent of Americans eat breakfast in the car on the way to work. Fifty percent of the meals we eat are consumed outside the home (USDA Dietary Survey). Of

Do You Want to Supersize That Lawsuit?

Move over tobacco industry. The new target of lawsuits is the ***fast-food industry.*** *Several suits filed against the major fast-food chains and food producers in 2003 alleged that fast food was making people fat and unhealthy. In one suit, a group of New York teenagers sued McDonald's, claiming the food made them obese. In another, an overweight man filed a class-action law suit against McDonald's, Burger King, Wendy's, and Kentucky Fried Chicken for jeopardizing his health. "They never explained to me what I was eating," said the plaintiff, Caesar Barber. Hmm.... Come on, let's take responsibility for what we put in our own mouths. We enjoy a fast-food burger and fries occasionally—but we don't make them a daily habit.*

course, eating fast food is a fun change once in a while. (By "fast food" or "junk food" we mean candy, chips and dip, fries, donuts—just about any food that contains a high amount of fat and calories.) Unfortunately it's a way of life for too many of us, and this convenience comes with a price. Junk food contributes hardly any nutritional value to the diet and provides excess calories and fat.

Supersize It

Not only do we eat too much junk food in America; we also eat more food than we need to fuel our bodies. We live in the age of "super-sized" portions. A study summarized in the *Journal of the American Medical Association* (Jan. 2003) reported that food portions had grown dramatically both at fast-food restaurants and at home. The average hamburger in 1977 was 5.7 ounces, and by 1996 the average size had grown to

Help Is on the Way

One of the nation's biggest food manufacturers, ***Kraft Foods,*** *is stepping up to the plate (pun intended) by changing its product recipes, reducing portions in some packages, and halting marketing to children at schools. It aims to produce more nutritional, "better-for-you" foods with lower salt, sugar, and fat contents. It has also pledged to offer smaller portion sizes. With Kraft making these changes, other food companies will likely follow its lead—resulting in healthier options for all of us. Right on!*

7 ounces, adding 100 extra calories. If you ask to supersize your fries, you add an extra 160 calories and 7 grams of fat to your meal.

She Should Live in Hershey, Pennsylvania

In the early 1980s, when the "more is better" training mentality ruled, ***Dave Scott,*** *a six-time winner of the grueling Ironman® Hawaii race, was reported to have rinsed his cottage cheese to remove the excess fat and salt. How times have changed!*

Today, ***Danelle Ballengee,*** *one of the best endurance athletes in the world and winner of every major adventure race, admits to being a big-time chocoholic and junk-food addict. She regularly consumes baking-size chocolate bars along with burgers and fries. According to Danelle, "It must be health food because it works for me." Genetics? Partly, but it's also because she leads a very active lifestyle.*

Just Right

- *1 ounce is the size of a matchbook (just right for a piece of cheese)*
- *2 tablespoons of peanut butter is the size of a golf ball*
- *½ cup of mashed potatoes or ice cream is the size of a tennis ball*
- *one serving of meat, poultry, or fish (3 ounces) is the size of a deck of cards*

All this excess adds up and we take in too many calories. If you consume more calories than you need for your daily activities, your body stores the extra calories as fat.

But exactly how many calories do we need each day? This depends on your body type, height, and level of activity. Here's a simple way to estimate your own daily caloric needs:

1. Divide your weight in pounds by 2.2 to get your weight in kilograms (calories are generally measured in kilograms).
2. Multiply your kilogram weight by one of the following:
   - Thirty if you are very active.
   - Twenty-five if you exercise three to four times per week.
   - Twenty if you are somewhat active (if you do housework, walk, or garden daily).

For example, a 130-pound female who is somewhat active would need roughly 1,200 calories to maintain her current weight.

Assessing Your Relationship with Food

Eating nutritiously is often a challenge because most of us simply don't have a healthy relationship with food. We all have triggers

Do the Math

These Web sites have excellent calculator programs that can help you get a handle on your daily food intake. Some let you gauge how many calories you need every day by using information about your height, weight, age, and activity level. Others help you calculate the amount of calories, proteins, and nutrients in the food you eat.

- *Nutrition Analysis Tools and System*
  http://nat.crgq.com
- *The Diet Channel*
  www.thedietchannel.com/diettools.htm
- *Calorie Control*
  www.caloriecontrol.org/calcalcs.html
- *iVillage*
  www.ivillage.com/diet

that make us want to eat: the smell of coffee brewing in the morning, the McDonald's hamburger ad on TV. But those triggers aren't always related to hunger. Eating plays a central role in our family and social lives, and we often turn to food for comfort when we're feeling stressed, bored, or excited. Perhaps you get a yen to eat chocolate when you're depressed, or tend to eat nonstop when you're nervous.

So how can you make your relationship with food healthier? First, you need to understand your physical and emotional relationship with food. Identifying food triggers can help you learn to avoid them and begin to get control of your eating. Experts recommend keeping a food diary for a week, recording what you eat, how much, and when, as well as how you feel at the time. Keeping a food log will help you identify the habits you can begin to change. Eventually, you'll eat when you're hungry and won't when you're not.

The No-Fries Tour

*As for us, we admit that road trips bring out our worst eating habits. We're hardly out of town before we find ourselves at the gas station, where **Barry** loads up on DOTS gumdrops and **Liz** digs in to a bag of M&Ms. But in 2002, we began an eight-city speaking tour for the sports retailer REI that we laughingly nicknamed "The No-Fries Tour."*

The humor worked and we remained fry-free and food-conscious for the entire three weeks we were on the road. Of course, Barry insisted on a "farewell-to-fries" bag of spuds the night before the tour started.

If you know your key times for snacking and overeating, try to schedule something for that time so you will stay busy. When we're on a road trip, sometimes we're smart and remember to pack a small cooler with healthy munchies like baby carrots. Here are some examples of nutritious snacks:

- fruit (fresh, dried, or frozen)
- fruit smoothies made with low-fat yogurt
- raw vegetables
- whole-grain cereals
- whole-grain crackers
- low-fat bean dips or salsa
- pretzels and rice cakes
- popcorn without butter
- frozen fruit popsicles
- low-fat cookies such as vanilla wafers, gingersnaps, and animal crackers

Start slowly, changing one element of your pattern at a time until it becomes a habit before adjusting anything else. Trying to change everything at once, for most people,

Does It Matter When I Eat?

There has been a lot of discussion over the years about whether it makes a difference what time you eat. Generally, it doesn't. If you eat an extra 1,000 calories in the morning, it's still an extra 1,000 calories—it really comes down to the total calories consumed. That said, here are some tips that might help you minimize the number of calories you take in every day:

- *Eat small amounts throughout the day. This helps keep the blood sugar level even, which is likely to prevent a binge later in the day.*
- *Eat a good breakfast every morning.*
- *Don't eat just before bedtime. This is when your metabolism is slowest, meaning it's more likely to store those calories as fat.*
- *Eat after exercise, when your metabolism is revved up.*

doesn't work. It takes several weeks before changes will become permanent—be patient. Over time, small changes lead to big changes.

Increase Your Metabolism

Everyone's metabolism, or their body's ability to transform food into fuel, is different. A lucky few born with a fast metabolism burn calories quickly and efficiently, instead of storing them as fat.

But there are some patterns that occur throughout the population. Metabolism rates do slow down as we get older—significantly for women after menopause. They also drop if we engage in restrictive dieting; that is, if the body does not get enough fuel, it conserves fuel by slowing the rate at which it burns calories. On the other hand, strength training and exercise can speed up your metabolism, because these activities replace fat with lean muscle, and lean muscle uses more energy than fat. While these activities don't increase your metabolism much, physical activity can help.

The bottom line is, get moving. If you run your car through the carwash rather than washing it yourself, if you pick up dinner at the drive-through on the way home rather than cook (usually more healthfully) at home; if you call the neighbor kid to come rake the leaves rather than raking them yourself, you'll never lose weight! More importantly, you won't be fit. Rev up those engines and get going!

A Great Cookbook

*One cookbook that we love and use often is **Family Circle Eat What You Love & Lose: Quick and Easy Diet Recipes from Our Test Kitchen** (2003). It contains over 250 delicious low-calorie recipes using everyday ingredients. And the recipes are easy—anyone can follow them. Give them a try!*

Getting a Jump-Start

The ultimate goal is to make good nutrition your normal approach to eating. But sometimes we just need a kick in the butt to get going. Need to lose weight? Just want to focus on your nutrition fitness?

There are a million ways to kick things off. Whenever Liz wants to lose a few pounds and get back on her nutrition track, she fires up a computer software program called Diet Power (for more information, log onto **www.dietpower.com**) to track everything she eats for a few days. Just this simple act reminds her how much she's really eating, and how much her body actually needs. The program allows users to input information on the exercise they do, and it continuously calculates individual metabolism based on calories eaten, exercise, and weight loss.

Some people swear by a jump-start using the Atkins Diet, or programs sold by Weight

Watchers, Jenny Craig, and others. Liz occasionally substitutes a Slim-Fast French vanilla shake for lunch each day for a week or two to get going. Following a prescribed diet for a few weeks can get you on the way to sustained weight loss.

Diets can be self-defeating since the weight lost is so often regained, plus some. But if you use the diet to kick-start your new lifestyle of eating better and exercising more—and you've checked with your doctor to let him/her know what you are doing—then it may be just the ticket. Following a two-week diet plan that an expert has put together for you can result in immediate weight loss and provide a great incentive to continue making positive changes.

Do eating and nutrition have to be a struggle? Please don't count every calorie, weigh every piece of food, or look up its glycemic index. Just eat consciously, include

Shopping Tips

- *Never shop when you're hungry. You'll buy too much, and too much of the wrong things. If you need a snack, eat an apple or banana on the way to the store.*
- *Choose low-fat foods. Read the labels carefully.*
- *Make a list of the things you need before going to the grocery store and then follow it strictly.*
- *Go to the produce section first and fill your basket with fruit and vegetables.*
- *Select non fat or low-fat desserts and sweets. Try angel food cake or ginger-snap cookies, vanilla wafers, or fig bars.*

plenty of variety, and eat reasonable portions. It's simple, really.

Learning to read food labels will help you make healthier food choices. The food label is a reliable, user-friendly source of valuable nutrition information—if you know how to read it.

Each label gives the U.S. Dietary Guidelines and the U.S. Daily Recommended Intake for healthy eating. The label lists the amount of calories, fat, fiber, and sugar in the food, as well as the percentage of key nutrients like calcium, iron, and sodium.

The information on nutrition labels is based on standardized portion sizes. These portions are intended to describe foods in commonly consumed amounts. Pay attention to the portion size—many people neglect to do this and end up consuming excess calories.

Laying Claim to Health

- *Fat free means the food has less than 0.5 grams of fat per serving.*
- *Low-fat means less than 3 grams of fat per serving.*
- *Cholesterol free means less than 2 mg per serving.*
- *Low cholesterol means less than 20 mg per serving.*
- *Low sodium means under 140 mg per serving.*
- *Low calorie means less than 40 calories per serving.*
- *Sugar free means less than 0.5 grams per serving.*
- *Fortified means the food provides more than 10 percent of the daily requirement for that nutrient.*

The Basics of Balance

What exactly is a balanced diet? One that provides all the nutrients needed, including carbohydrates, protein, and fats. It also provides the vitamins, minerals, fiber, and fluids necessary to maintain health without weight gain or loss.

Carbohydrates supply energy to the body and maintain normal blood glucose (sugar) levels. The highest concentration of carbohydrates is found in whole grains and cereals, but they are also found in fruits, vegetables, and dairy products. Most of the fuel you use while active is derived from carbohydrates.

Protein helps make muscle and ensures normal immune response and maintains enzyme action in the body. Protein comes from animal products, including meat, poultry, and dairy products. Fish also provides a good source of protein, as do some plant foods, such as legumes and soy beans. A healthy percentage of protein in your diet averages from 20 to 30 percent of your total caloric intake.

Fats are essential for maintaining the structure and support of our organs. Although fat should be limited in our diet, it is important to eat some dietary fat each day to ensure good health. Fat is obtained from many sources—meats, dairy products, and plants such as nuts, seeds, coconut, and avocado.

Food labels break down the food's fat content into the categories of saturated,

A Calorie by Any Other Name ... Is Still a Calorie

Low fat doesn't always mean low calorie. When it comes to maintaining or losing weight, it's the total number of calories consumed per day that counts ... and only the number of calories. Low fat is good, but not if the total number of calories consumed increases as a result.

Eat the Rainbow Every Day

Try to create a colorful plate of food at every meal—chances are you'll be eating a healthy balanced diet. Include the blues and purples in eggplant and blueberries, the reds of radishes and tomatoes, the yellows of squash and citrus fruits, and the deep greens in kale and broccoli. A rainbow of colors on your plate helps to ensure you're getting adequate vitamins, nutrients, and minerals.

polysaturated, and monosaturated fat. This information can help you choose food low in total fat. It also makes it possible to select foods that contain monosaturated fat—the "healthiest" fat.

As part of your new active lifestyle, remember to increase the amount of water you drink each day. Many people are chronically

Drink to Your Health

Fill a container with the equivalent of eight glasses of water (64 ounces) and keep it in the refrigerator. Drink the entire contents every day and refill the container at night before going to bed. That way you' ll ensure that you' ve drunk enough water.

dehydrated, which can cause mild headaches, as well as fatigue. Drink a minimum of eight to ten glasses (that hold eight ounces) of water every day. The bigger you are, the more you should drink.

Keep snacks simple, keep meals colorful. Pay attention to what you eat, when you eat, and why you eat. Try to eat consciously and with intention. You'll be healthier for it!

Conclusion

We can change. All of us have the power to reverse the downward trend of fitness by starting with ourselves. It only requires a willingness to try a new approach to fitness—one that simply focuses on being more active and having fun rather than an expensive gym membership, hours of boring "workout" drudgery, or jumping on the latest diet bandwagon. You can forget the 70's running craze, the 80's "feel the burn" craze, and the 90's hardcore gym craze.... It's time to rediscover your true nature through moving and having fun.

The examples in this book have inspired others to find and enjoy fitness. It is our hope that you will begin to increase the amount of activity in your life by doing things you enjoy, even if they don't fit into the traditional definition of exercise. Take the first step to get yourself movin' and groovin'—who knows where it will lead? The first step is usually the hardest, but you can make it easier by doing things that make you laugh, feel peaceful, and get energized. Remember to play.

Being fit is easier than you have been led to believe. If fitness is fun, it will become ingrained in your lifestyle. In no time you will begin to feel better, look forward to your activities, and reap the rewards of good health. Once you get the hang of it, we are sure you will begin looking for even more ways to have fun. There is no end to the ideas ... and we'd love to hear what activities inspire you, so we can pass them on to others!

Liz & Barry

www.fitandfunforlife.com